The Y. A. K. Diet

Why weight loss diets work, why they don't work,

And a new approach.

B.B. Stryke

Table of Contents

The Y.A.K Diet Introduction

Part One

Chapter One - Background 8
Chapter Two - Why diet books are written 10
Chapter Three - The "secret" 13
Chapter Four - The diet book formula 16
Chapter Five - Why diet books books don't work 20
Chapter Six - Why diet books do work 23
Chapter Seven - A new way of thinking 26
Chapter Eight - Be responsible for your own 27
      actions

Part Two

Chapter Nine - The Y.A.K diet 31
Chapter Ten - How do I start the Y.A.K diet? 33
Chapter Eleven - How do you lose weight? 35
Chapter Twelve - What foods should I eat? 37
Chapter Thirteen - I deserve a treat 48
Chapter Fourteen - Can I replace this food with 51
      that food?
Chapter Fifteen - The G. G. 53
Chapter Sixteen - Final thoughts 55

Introduction

Before I launch into the details, I need to clarify that there are several definitions of the word "diet". It could mean just the food you are currently eating, it could mean weight gain or weight loss. In general, in this little book, I am thinking about weight loss, then ongoing target weight stability for… ever! However the general principles are similar however you define the word.

Ok here we go with yet another diet book, but this time I am convinced that my new, revolutionary, approach will work! I consider myself to be fairly intelligent. I am a qualified accountant, man of the world. Good at trivia quizzes. Not genius material by a longshot, but I do know how many beans make 5. However despite all my knowledge, I am overweight. I have read quite a few diet books over the years and generally take an interest in food and ingredients. I think I understand the basics of how the different food groups affect the body. But guess what? I'm still fat! A few days ago

I got the Times newspaper and one of the headlines on one of the supplements was "Reviewed inside, the latest summer diets". Obviously I was intrigued.

One of them may be the magic bullet I have been looking for all of my life. I then had a mini epiphany. Do I really need to absorb more knowledge about any new diet, or new ways to lose weight? Surely after 60 odd years on the planet (Earth) and with reasonable intelligence, I should already know all I need to know about why I am overweight and what to do about it. The germ of an idea for a revolutionary diet book was born. You hold the result in your hands.

The book is written in two parts.

Part One - A review of why diets work and don't work, the problem with diet plans, diet books and the diet "industry".

Part Two - My new revolutionary approach to dieting to get to your target weight without jargon, bizarre "special" ingredients and instead a concentrated, foolproof method that gives you the tools that you need to lose weight once and for all. Aka "The Y.A.K. Diet"

PART ONE – BACKGROUND

Chapter One

Why diet books are written

Diet books are written in order to help overweight people lose weight right? Maybe! I think diet books are largely written to sell copy and make money for the author and publisher. Of course all parties want the book to be successful as the more copies sold, the greater the profit. If any particular diet takes off there will be major profits to be made. Look at the success of the F Plan, or the Atkins diet a few years ago – major best sellers. The sale of the original book can be lucrative but of course follow up items such as "Book No. 2", recipes, vegetarian version, tours, talks, videos, TV chat shows and fame will likely follow! Nothing wrong with any of that of course but will all that help you lose weight? I doubt it. The reason you are buying these books is to lose weight but that is not the same reason the book was written! The authors may be genuine in their desire to see people lose weight. I am genuine too. For a diet to be successful the author would want many many people to claim that their particular diet works which of course

increases popularity of the diet and hence further sales and

fame.

Chapter Two

Diet book authors

Most diet books are written by "experts" in the field. The most obvious expert is a Doctor. If you can get a Doctor prefix to your name, the perceived authority to write a diet book is immense. If you are a doctor you must know what you are talking about! This is irrespective of what your actual Doctorate is in. I expect if you were a Doctor of Theology you could write a diet book and no one would question your credentials to write a diet book. See for example recent famous Doctors who have written diet books (will not name names!). If you cannot be a Doctor, then you will have to settle for the next tier down – i.e. "Nutritionist".

As far as I can see nutrition is a subject that can be studied and I'm sure it is very interesting – the effect that different foodstuffs have on the body: vitamins, minerals etc. Does that make you qualified to write a diet book? Well maybe but that is no guarantee of talking sense. But the title of

Nutritionist does conjure up some level of authority, i.e. I know what I am talking about and you plebs should listen to me!

If you cannot be a Doctor or a Nutritionist, then next level down is either a journalist or a cookery writer – e.g. a Health Writer for a newspaper or magazine. True, a trained journalist in that field may have some knowledge of what they are writing about, a cookery writer or chef will have knowledge about food. They will certainly have the skills to express themselves in a persuasive way, but particular skills to write a diet book that can consistently be followed to successfully lose weight – forget it!

Worst of the worst in my pecking order for "expertise" is the Celebrity. A totally meaningless endorsement but somehow in this celebrity obsessed day and age, if a diet book is "written" by a celebrity, accompanied of course by before and after pictures, it is a recipe for success. No idea why but it works time and time again. We see celebrities on the T.V.

and I suppose we identify with them to some extent. If they have lost weight and swear by a particular diet then why wouldn't we want to be like them?

So to complete the hierarchy of credentials' who am I? I'm a 60 odd year male retired Accountant who is a bit overweight —way down the pecking order of diet book author credentials.

Chapter Three

The "secret"

For any diet book to be successful (note this is not the same thing as any <u>diet</u> to be successful!) there must be some sort of new knowledge or technique which the author, in his or her infinite wisdom, has just discovered and is willing to share with you. Of course scientific knowledge is increasing all the time so there is of course genuine new knowledge being discovered or proved. If you look back at TV adverts from, say, 50 years ago smoking was good for you! As scientific knowledge improves and pushes human knowledge forward, there is no reason to doubt that what was once considered sensible dietary advice is now not sensible – and vice versa. It is therefore correct to assume that new dietary advice should be made available to the public - and why not in a diet book? However, having said all that, it is clear that most diet books have a secret to share – and it's a more often than not a load of rubbish, but written is such a way that it sounds like it could/should work. Here are some recent examples…

1) Eating normally on some days, but restricted on others (5:2 diet)
2) Calorie counting
3) Low Carbohydrates
4) Not eating certain foods after, say, 7.00 pm
5) Diets based on certain lifestyles, e.g. Mediterranean or French diet.

The point is that any new diet book must say something new – otherwise you may as well keep publishing the same book over and over again. If there is nothing new to say why bother saying it! Of course, changes of publishing style, e.g. font, photos and celebrity endorsement can make old news look new but the point is that each new diet book must promise and promote some "secret" or new news that up to now has not been made available to you, the great overweight public.

The "secret" that is disclosed in the mass of diet books may of course be good or bad. Many many books contain sensible advice about types of food to either eat or avoid – and when to eat or not eat them. However a lot of them are complete rubbish and are either dangerous nutritionally or almost impossible to follow. My diet has no secret. It is based on sensible tried and tested advice… but more of the Y.A.K. diet later.

Chapter Four

The diet book formula

Read any diet book and they invariable follow this formula:

1) Credentials of the author – in other words why you should follow his or her advice.

2) The "science" behind the secret – why other diets fail and why this particular one won't.

3) Case studies of "normal people" who have followed the diet and had amazing results.

4) How and why the diet works on a physiological level.

5) Lists of foods either to eat or avoid – plus where you can buy any "magic" ingredients.

6) Before the diet – measure your weight, BMI etc. Plan your goals and motivation.

7) The classic line of "see your doctor before embarking on this diet" – to me, if you need to see your doctor before embarking on a diet there must be something not right about the diet. E.g. restriction of certain food groups. If

you are eating and drinking sensibly there surely should be no need to see a Doctor beforehand – and how many people do so anyway? I have tried loads of diets over the years and never bothered seeing a Doctor beforehand.

8) Frequently asked question – of course carefully selected by the author!

9) What to buy and why you should clear out your cupboards – in other words throw away good, expensive food you have previously bought, and replace with a new list of food that if the diet is correctly followed, will cause weight loss.

10) A 14 day "cleanse" part of the diet – why do they always do this? Well I know why, so you can see immediate results that encourages you to continue and allows you to claim that this diet is brilliant!

11) A month long "continuing plan", where you are allowed to eat a bit more than the 14 day plan. This is usually because the 14 day bit is so restrictive that there is zero chance of continuing so they allow you to eat a larger

variety of "treats" so you stay with the plan a bit longer before it all goes pear shaped (same as you!).

12) Maintenance program – after the month long bit this is where you again introduce larger helpings, or some previously restricted foods. I read this part of the diet as the "where it all goes wrong and you put weight back on" bit.

13) Tips to help you when you eat out (parties, buffets etc.)

14) Appendices with tables of which foods you should buy and eat in order to follow the "magic rules" – possibly with either calories, food points, Glycemic Index values or whatever.

15) Finally, there is usually at least half the book comprising either a complete list of meals for the 14 day "clean" section – e.g. Day 8 snack you can have a 7 Almonds! (And see the Appendix for a list of expensive suppliers!) Followed by lists of recipes split into sections of breakfasts, lunch, evening meals, snacks, drinks or whatever.

I would like to suggest that, however well-intentioned the potential dieter is, no one is really going to follow all this. There are many reasons for failure, but in truth how many people actually follow the particular diet to the letter? The good news for the author of course is that the diet is not the issue, the problem is that people have not followed it correctly – for the author it's a win win situation. If you follow the diet to the letter you will lose weight. If you don't – it's your fault!

A few years ago I was following some diet plan. It listed recipes to follow exactly to the letter for 14 days. Day 1, Meal 1 I was missing one of the ingredients. So I substituted for another one. See the problem? I failed at the first hurdle, and it was my fault not the diets. In reality this sort of restricted plan in unworkable.

Chapter Five

Why diet books don't work

These are the main reasons that diet books <u>don't</u> work.

1) You have to spend a lot of money filling your cupboard and fridge with lots of "special" possibly expensive ingredients from hard to find locations or websites.

2) You have to follow their rules to the letter which can be a burden both financially, socially and a time burden. – Who wants to spend 3 hours each night preparing special meals?

3) It is very difficult to follow any plan for any significant length of time – we are only human so our resolve weakens over time. Also what happens after you finish the plan? We all know the feeling of slipping. It's not great is it the feeling of failure but us seasoned dieters know the impact failure can have. Why do we put ourselves through it? Our friends and families, however supportive they are, don't always want to hear about our

latest diet, or our latest failures do they? – Boring! (Especially if they are thin and wonder what the fuss is all about!)

4)   We generally have short attention spans (and getting shorter if you believe the media) – what? Have you read this far?? It's easy to lose a bit of weight on a new diet, think we have cracked it then immediately allow ourselves some treats ("I deserve a treat") and hey presto… the weight magically reappears and we claim the diet was rubbish and quietly forgot we were ever really on it!

5)   The "rules" of the particular diet we are following do not fit into our lifestyle. A good example of this is social situations. However careful I am about my eating, if I go to someone's house for a meal, it's rude not to stuff your face after they have gone to all that trouble of cooking isn't it?

6)   Most of us seasoned dieters regularly kid ourselves that we are on a diet, but the evidence is that we are not – If you have ever seen the Secret Eaters T.V. program

where fat people claim they hardly eat anything but never lose weight, hidden cameras suggest that they eat rubbish all day long and are either in denial or "forget" to count it in their diet. E.g. tasting food when cooking, eating your kids leftovers, forgetting to count the odd biscuit when washing up etc. etc.

Chapter Six

Why diet books do work

These are the main reasons diet books <u>do</u> work.

1) You will be following a plan. By definition if you are following a diet plan – pretty much to the letter – you will lose weight because you are not eating as much as usual. Every diet plan works by restriction. You will have picked a particular diet as you believe it will fit in with your lifestyle, or it has been recommended by friends or the media. You will (initially) lose weight too as you are keen to follow the plan to the letter and will be thinking about your food and restricting yourself in some way.

2) If you are following a plan you will be thinking about what you eat. Even with the occasional slippage you will definitely be eating less than normal so will lose weight.

3) Some of the diet books/plans will certainly be accurate in their message and not just gimmicks. It certainly is possible to eat normal healthy food, not feel hungry, and lose weight. I do however believe that many of the faddy diets are either nutritionally unsound or just too difficult to follow over a sustained period. Even if the diet is a gimmick you will lose weight initially as you are following a plan.

4) Whatever diet plan you follow, you will certainly learn some skills and knowledge about food, food groups, tips and recipes that may help you. You may even learn some emotional skills about, for example, why you overeat, what are the trigger points, emotional and psychological reasons for overeating. Knowledge is never a bad thing so following a diet plan, and learning how it works – or is supposed to work – will help you in your general knowledge about dieting. However I always think of the maxim "All the gear and no idea". I consider myself reasonably intelligent. I am a qualified accountant. I know quite a lot about food groups and the

effect they have on the body. But guess what? I'm still overweight and have been for years. Therefore, my "intelligence" and food knowledge built up over the years is as much use as a chocolate teapot and has not helped me at all.

Chapter Seven

A new way of thinking

All of the above chapters have been my attempt to persuade you that following any particular diet book or plan is never going to work. Yes it may work for a short while, and for a few special people may be the help they need to lose weight permanently. But for most of us we know, deep down, that it isn't going to last. We will face yet another failure, feel terrible that we are failures and cheese off our friends and family. What then is the secret to losing weight forever? What is the diet plan? Where are the pages and pages of recipe ideas to follow? What is my "secret" knowledge that I am willing to impart to you fellow tubbies?

Chapter Eight

Be responsible for your own actions

In life, most of us are constantly looking for a quick fix to our problems. Life these days is increasingly busy – despite all the fantastic labour saving devices we have, we seem to have busier lives than ever before. This can make it difficult to concentrate on a long term, major, life changing course of action. Weight loss is a great example of this. To help us, we are often looking for help. That help can come in the form of, say, all the family losing weight together, joining a weight loss club, having a personal trainer or setting weight loss goals. It can be very difficult going at it alone and of course I do understand the need many people have to reach out and get help. We seasoned dieters know how hard it is, and in fact how boring it is, to be constantly thinking about what you can or can't eat and how long it will be until the next meal – it's awful. I am certainly not recommending that you avoid any third party assistance (like losing weight with a buddy).

However – deep down, outside pressure and influence is not the thing that matters, it has to come from within. I urge you all to try to develop your own skills in the way you tackle your weight loss. Take responsibility and do not abdicate responsibility to anyone else. You need to go it alone. No one is saying it is easy. I think naturally slim people do not realise how hard it can be. I have heard naturally slim people say stuff like "I was so busy at work I forgot to have lunch"! What? How can you forget a meal!?

The worry of relying on others too much is this. When the party is over and you have achieved your goal, guess what? The weight piles back on. You have let everyone down. You have to go at it alone and learn your weak points, learn tools to overcome the hiccups on the road. You cannot rely on anyone else – they all have their own problems you know and cannot be as invested in you, as you are!

In the same vein, I would not trust celebrities, nutritionists, food manufacturers or celebrity chefs. They do not have your best interests at heart – only theirs. Make your own mind up, Make your own judgements. Find out the facts yourself, no need to rely on others to do it for you. Trust yourself. You are unique … just like everyone else!

I do realise the irony of dismissing the entire concept of diet books and urging you to ignore the whole diet industry - by writing a diet book! Bonkers I know, but how else can I get the information to you guys!

Next section is the "How to do it" bit.

PART TWO – THE Y.A.K. DIET

Chapter Nine

The Y. A. K. diet

Firstly let's clear up what Y.A.K. means. Nothing to do with the woolly mammal but means…

You Already Know

As you, the reader, has bought this little book, I assume you are intelligent, reasonably well adjusted, erudite, well read and interested in this subject! Therefore I have no worries that you cannot follow the basic philosophy of the Y.A.K diet. The idea is that it is extremely likely that you already know what food is good or bad for you, the quantities you should be eating and when you should be eating. Use the knowledge you already have with your own common sense to reach your weight loss goal.

Do you need to know that eating a takeaway every night is good for you or bad for you? Do you need to know that having four slices of jam on toast for breakfast is good or bad for you? Deep down, and perhaps not even that deep, you already know you shouldn't be eating it. You do not need a diet book, or diet plan, to tell you what you can or can't eat – YOU ALREADY KNOW if you think about it.

Chapter Ten

How do I start the Y.A.K diet?

Good news…You have just started! Start now, immediately. No need for a medical, or to clean your cupboards out, or to buy any special food. Each minute of each day is time you could spend losing weight rather than thinking about doing it, therefore why delay starting? You do not need to have a big build up to gather momentum, just go for it right now. In the past I have said things like "I'm going away for the weekend so will start my diet on Monday, or after the holidays" etc. Load of rubbish – why prevaricate – just get on with it!

Any obstacles in the way of you starting your diet now will be there for the rest of your life. For example "I'm going out for a meal tonight so may as well start in the morning". Ok then so, after tonight, when you're allegedly "on the diet" you will never go out for a meal again? The temptation and excuses are all around you so no reason to put it off – Start

NOW!

34

Chapter Eleven

How do you lose weight?

You lose weight by doing the following:

1) Eating less food.

2) Exercising more.

3) Eating less food and exercising more.

4) All three!

Simples!

Brief paragraph on exercise – Any reasonable exercise will be beneficial to your health in general, and your weight loss journey in particular. I'm not particularly going to talk about exercise here, but whatever your age or current fitness levels, some physical activity will be beneficial. In line with the Y.A.K philosophy, you don't need to spend any money on this – open your door and go for a walk! It will get air into your lungs, stretch and loosen your muscles and joints, increase your metabolism and improve your mood! I'd always keep it simple – you need a lifetime of good habits based on the Y.A.K approach so – walking, gardening, housework, sex, frisbee! (Not necessarily all at the same time.)

Unless you are a serious athlete with specific food needs for your training regime, for most of us, exercise will certainly help you but the main way to lose weight will be to eat less food. Probably a lot less. YOU ALREADY KNOW this.

Let's quietly think sensibly about losing weight. Whichever diet rules you are following, you know that you will have to eat a lot less food than you do now. The emphasis should be on eating less rather than following a particular plan. You know deep down it's not going to be easy. Any small increase in exercise will not be enough to help us lose weight. Eating less food – and certainly less of rubbish food is the answer.

Chapter Twelve

What foods should I eat?

The most sensible advice is to eat healthy whole foods and cut out the crap! Just eat less of it.

You have taken a chance on me by buying this book, I am taking a chance on you by trusting that YOU ALREADY KNOW what is good or bad for you.

Nutrition is a big subject. Some knowledge of the subject will certainly be beneficial in your weight loss journey but you do not need to be "world nutrition champion" though to be aware of the basics. (Is that a thing?) To explain the basics, in general, avoid take-away, ready meals and highly processed food.

Two general rules of thumb.

1) The more ingredients in a food – the worse it is for you.

2) If you can't pronounce or spell any of the ingredients – it will not be good for you.

All commonsense diets and sensible current knowledge will say roughly the following…

1) Lots of fresh fruit and vegetables.

2) Little meat and fish, little dairy foods.

3) Low or no amounts of man-made processed rubbish – less sugar, white flour & rice and so on.

In other words eat mostly plants and as unprocessed as possible. Avoid man made snacks, convenience food, regular fast food and take-aways. Added sugar. Avoid crap! But YOU ALREADY KNOW this don't you?

In the words of the US author Michael Pollan…

Eat food. Not too much. Mostly plants.

The hardest part of any diet is not what foods I can or can't eat, but just getting out of the habit of eating so much of the stuff – just decide you're going to eat less quantity and seriously cut down on the stuff. YOU ALREADY KNOW this.

You have to think that every time you put some food in your mouth, you are making a decision. The decision is "will eating this help me on my diet?" There is no such thing as negative calories so in truth every single mouthful of food will add to your weight gain. However of course, we do have to eat to stay alive and no one is suggesting you should fast. But you must realise that you need to cut down in order to lose weight. You need to get in the habit of asking yourself "How will eating this bag of crisps/chips (family size) help me lose weight?" I am sure anyone of any intelligence level will know the answer.

For example, you go out with the family for a meal. While you are looking through the menus and deciding what to eat the waiter asks if you want some bread and olives while you are waiting. What for??

You order a starter – what's all that about? A mini meal before you eat your main meal?

You order your main meal and the waiter asks if you want any sides – why? To accompany my big main meal I am ordering side dishes with extra food on?

Of course by then you are stuffed but the Desert menu arrives and you find yourself ordering a pudding – YOU ALREADY KNOW it's wrong! How do you feel after scoffing all that? If you are like me you will feel terrible and think "I've done it again. Got carried away and had too much. I'll definitely start the diet tomorrow!"

Years ago I went for a curry after work with the "Lads" from work. My mate told me this…

"Have 1 or 2 poppadoms, never order a starter, never order a desert, only have a main curry meal with either rice or naan – never both. Ideally share the rice with a friend".

It's true you know. Have you ever had 2 or more poppadoms, eaten a starter then the waiter arrives with his trolley full of food and you think to yourself "I'm not actually hungry anymore". It's so easy to get carried away and over order when you are hungry, and with other people. Resist the temptation and stick to the plan. After the meal you will be nicely content and full without being over stuffed!

Mrs. Stryke and I now do this. We will have 1 poppadom each, a main curry type dish each and share 1 portion of either rice or naan bread. Guess what? It's enough and you feel great afterwards. Think through this concept with your own meals out and try not to get caught up in the frenzy of over ordering just because you are hungry.

Don't forget that restaurants, cafes, pubs etc. are very good at selling you a dream about all the food you can eat. Beautifully printed menus, nice atmosphere, serving staff asking if you need any sides or specials etc. You need to be aware of the tricks and be on your guard. They are not your friends!

The other thing to be aware of are special diet foods. If they are branded as diet foods they will probably have low levels of either calories, sugar (same thing), fat or "points". I suggest to you that it will be crapola of the highest order. For it to taste acceptable the loss of, for example, sugar, will be compensated by either man-made sugar derivatives or higher levels of salt or fat to make it taste acceptable. People kid themselves that it is healthy and doing them some good –

here is the news…it 'aint and guess what?? YOU ALREADY KNOW! It's a money making industry, nothing more. Manufacturers don't care about you, only their profits. Be true to yourself and eat good quality whole food. Don't abdicate responsibility to anyone else (especially food manufacturers,) be in charge of your own body, your own diet and your own goals.

Here is a good example of processed rubbish masquerading as healthy – rice cakes. If you look at a typical packet it is claimed to be low in fat. Low according to who? Low relative to what? Is it low in good fat or bad fat? Hmm it tastes nice so where does that nice taste come from? Could it be processed white sugar? Is there a lot of salt in it? Is the actual rice any good or is it bleached to death cheapo white rice with zero nutrients? Perhaps it's cheaper for them to manufacture it using bleached white rice but don't worry – they have added a load of vitamins and minerals to replace the ones washed away in the manufacturing process. Eh? What? You get the idea I'm sure. Just say you are following a low calorie diet and the rice cakes claim to be low calorie. That makes it ok now as complies with my low calorie diet plan. YOU ALREADY KNOW it is rubbish. Pack it in and just eat good quality whole food but less of it. Trust me I have had years of kidding myself about this sort of thing. Don't waste your money on special diet food – eat normal fresh whole food but less of it.

In writing this little book I have thought long and hard about what sort of guidance to put in regarding what and what not to eat. You have probably realised by now that there is very little actual advice here. If I was to create a long list of do's and don'ts that will negate the whole point of the book. I will certainly have missed out some items. Also what are the chances of you keeping the list with you… forever? Zilch! The Y.A.K. concept means you already know the rules and you have to adapt and be aware of them every time you eat. You are the best judge and YOU ALREADY KNOW what is right and wrong.

When hungry (or when you think you are hungry) it is so easy to get carried away, over order, make too much (portion sizes) and generally get carried away. One thing I have been trying to do recently is order or make a small amount. Eat it with the thought in my head that "If I am still hungry later I can have something else". Guess what? You are not hungry later. I find that once I clear my plate my thought process is as follows…

1) Cor that was nice. Is there any more?
2) I might have a bit more later
3) Come to think of it I am nicely satisfied, not hungry anymore but also not stuffed.

Try it when you are eating next. It does work.

When I was a young lad at home, we would always have a large pudding immediately after our main meal, (Apple pie with custard etc.) With regards to the Y.A.K. diet that is obviously a no no, but some sort of healthy fruit type thing could of course be suitable. Mrs. Stryke has the best idea by saying "I may have a sweet later". When later comes you may decide not to bother once you have overcome the frenzy of eating, or have a small piece of fruit or whatever. My attitude from when I was younger was "I want pudding now!" It is clearly not a good idea, so if you abstain for a while and let the eating frenzy die down you can then sensibly think of your correct, Y.A.K. inspired decision.

As you go through each day, you are surrounded by temptation. It can be a combination of clever marketing by fast food restaurants, eating at a friend's house ("go on have a pudding"), working at home with the infamous lure of the biscuit tin. You have to be on your guard all day every day. You can of course argue that, say, one little biscuit with a cup of tea mid-morning will not be bad for me. The answer is of course it may not hinder you too much – but keep asking yourself these questions...

Do I need it? Do I want it? And…will eating this biscuit help me lose weight?

It's pretty obvious what the answer is. Distract yourself with something else. Don't fall into the trap of having a treat. Having a treat is usually what you say to yourself when you know you are eating something you shouldn't. How do you feel after the treat? Terrible I imagine. Don't succumb, be strong and think of the goal of losing weight and the great feeling of knowing that you have mentally overcome the obstacle.

Chapter Thirteen

I deserve a treat

We all kid ourselves all the time in many ways – how are you at driving a car? Above average I expect – same as me. Funny how we are all above average and kid ourselves - but especially with food if you are carrying a bit of excess weight. Here are some examples of how we kid ourselves…

1) Friday night, working all week, don't want to cook – "let's get a takeaway"

2) Went to friends for a meal – felt I had to eat the pudding as they made it especially.

3) There was only three biscuits left so made sense to eat them all and then throw the packet out. I have been very clever and removed the temptation. Well true I ate them but I'm not going to throw expensive food away and there was only 3.

4) Birthday cakes brought into work.

5) Mrs. Stryke (slim) was eating crisps (chips). I wasn't hungry at all but suddenly found myself eating two packets to "join in the fun".

With all of these examples, and many other real life situations you have to constantly ask yourself the following question.

"How will eating this food help me in my goal to lose weight?

I think YOU ALREADY KNOW the answer.

Part of the problem of course is, life is too short to not occasionally enjoy yourself. And eating is certainly one of the great pleasures of life for most of us. The social side of eating together is also very important as part of life's happiness. Should I never eat, say, a birthday cake ever again? What is the answer?

The "official" answer is, of course, "Do not eat it", however in moderation these type of foods can be eaten but always think to yourself. "Eating this cake will not help me lose weight", and also be prepared for the lapse by deciding in advance what you will be having, and the consequences of your actions.

You should be thinking about not some sort of fad diet with list of "rules" but a sensible course of action for you to lose and maintain weight loss for the rest of your life. A few minor hiccups on the road will not be a problem but what is a problem is the concept of "I deserve a treat" which, as we all know, very soon slips into constant treats and ends up with you not actually dieting at all (but you will kid yourself you are dieting for a little while yet before giving up and then trying the next diet that comes your way).

Chapter Fourteen

Can I replace this food with that food?

One of the diet books I own has the ubiquitous FAQ section. It's a load of standard rubbish – carefully selected by the author, However there is one particular question and answer that I think about it all the time. Here is the question…

Q   "Can I eat low carb bars? I have heard that they might stall my weight loss"

Here is the published answer.

A.   "You can eat whatever you like"

I think that is a great answer. You can eat whatever you like. Can you see why I like that answer based on the Y.A.K diet? Every food you put in your mouth will have an impact on your diet and weight loss. You continually have to weigh up the consequences. Is the low carb bar a treat? Is it a meal replacement? Who knows? Who cares? Eat proper meals of natural foods but eat a lot less of it. Don't eat man-made rubbish.

Chapter Fifteen

The G. G.

In the town where I live is a juggling chap. I won't say his stage name but I'll call him The G.G. I have known him on and off for years and he is a very pleasant fellow. I took a night school course with him once years ago but I see him from time to time occasionally at local fetes etc. doing juggling courses for the kids. He is not very tall but was always a bit, well, "roundy".

Anyway, Mrs. Stryke and I were at a local carnival recently and I saw he had a stall. We went over to see him and he looked great. He had lost lots of weight – at least 2 stone (30 lbs.') I would estimate. Of course I eagerly told him he looked great and asked him his secret. This is what he said…

"Eat normal meals but less of it, no snacks and go out walking every evening"

There you go. It's the Y.A.K diet in a nutshell. Eat normal food, less of it. Don't snack on rubbish, and gently exercise on a regular basis. No counting points, carbs or calories. No expensive diet fads. No gyms or diet equipment. Simple, cheap and honest. And let me tell you the results were sensational. He did it, I can do it. You can do it!

Chapter Sixteen

Final thoughts

As mentioned in Part 1, you will not find in this book any recipes, diet plans, Q' and A's or lists of ingredients. All I have tried to do is critique diet books, diet fads and manufactured foods that are designed to do the work for you. If you think about it for a short while, people are generally lazy and want to abdicate dietary responsibility to someone else - e.g. a diet book, food manufacturer, a celebrity, the Government (5 a day anyone?). We all do this type of thinking all the time in all walks of life… "The council need to do something", or "The government should sort it out" or "God will save me". Learn to think for yourself and trust your own judgement. With regards to your body, your goals and your food choices, who do you think is best placed to make this decision? I'll give you a clue…it's not a celebrity who has written a diet book! Eat fresh unprocessed food, exercise more. There is no need to count points, calories, GI index, eat before 7.00pm or any of that rubbish.

You have a whole lifetime ahead of you to eat and drink and get on with your life. Eating and drinking is one of the many pleasures of life, but eating healthily, with sensible portions is obviously the best way forward. This little book's main point is to tell you that you already know the "rules" of what to eat. You don't need to learn any more of it. You just need to get on with it and to trust your own knowledge and judgement to decide what is best for you for the rest of your life. You will not, or cannot have this or any other book with you at all times to let you know the "rules". It is simply not workable. Trust yourself to take responsibility to make good choices and remember…

… You Already Know.